Angry Mind

Finding Peace in Your Life

Charles Lamont

Legal Disclaimer

The information contained in this book is strictly for educational purpose only. The content of this book is the sole expression and opinion of its author and not necessarily that of the publisher. It is not intended to cure, treat, and diagnose any kind of disease or medical condition. It is sold with the understanding that the publisher is not rendering any type of medical, psychological, legal, or any other kind of professional advice. You should seek the services of a competent professional before applying concepts in this book. Neither the publisher nor the individual author(s) shall be liable for any physical, psychological, emotional, financial, or commercial damages, directly or indirectly by the use of this material, which is provided "as is", and without warranties. Therefore, if you wish to apply ideas contained in this book, you are taking full responsibility for your actions.

Table of Contents

Introduction

Anger is one of the most common feelings experienced by human beings. As a matter of fact, feelings of annoyance, irritation and anger are emotions that are unavoidable because it is linked to the human nature. However, it is important to understand that anger comes with its own set of rigid beliefs and blinders. It not only narrows your thinking but also sets you in a cycle of blame game.

By covering its tracks, anger makes you absolutely certain that your view in a particular situation is 100 percent accurate. What makes matters worse is that any emotion you feel at the time when you are angry enhances the odds that next time you will feel the same emotion. Anger has insidious ways of controlling your mind, dominates your days and ultimately your life.

Anger, like any other negative emotion is part of our daily experiences and you do not necessarily have to become a victim of it. Psychological science makes it absolutely clear that the power to cultivate or prolong angry experiences is squarely in your hands. Anger does not have to become your lifestyle. Science has documented what anger can do when you allow it to become your baseline or first impulse. Among the things you stand to suffer include strained relationships, compromised health and unhappiness.

If anger has in one way or another come to rule and ruin your life, you have the opportunity to change all that and write a different script. This book can help you achieve that. It draws on ancient wisdom and 21st century breakthroughs to calm your angry mind. In it, you will learn the core practices of compassion and mindfulness as well as how and when to deploy them.

1: The Science of Mindfulness

In the words of Jose Ortega, "Tell me what you pay attention to and I will tell you who you are." Your thoughts do not represent and do not have to rule over you even when they indicate irritation, anger, blame or judgment. As a human being, your scope is wider, more complex and amazing than any of the thoughts that infiltrate your mind.

Every one of us is born with an innate capacity to be mindful. This means you have what you need to practice mindfulness even without external input. Mindfulness relies on your attentiveness in the present moment while you maintain an open heart. Fortunately, this is something every human being can do. Mindfulness is simply defined as pausing to pay attention on purpose and without judgment while gently noticing and simply being present with what is, at the moment.

Mindfulness is important as it helps release you from the inner momentum and over-identification of becoming something more in life. Being more mindful does not necessarily mean that you have to stop what you are doing, but rather making deliberate efforts not to be lost in your daily life. Mindfulness can make you discover new frontiers and possibilities where you live in ways that are not so busy yet more satisfying.

Learning how to rest in awareness, notice more carefully and remain present for the things that are here and now, will help you change your relationship to your feelings and thoughts in more liberating and remarkable ways. When you mindfully observe your interactions with the external world and the flow of your inner life, you will develop a deeper understanding of your emotions and thoughts. Remember emotions and thoughts such as scorn, hostility, dislike and anger are never your permanent identity. They are temporal and rely on each other as well as other temporal conditions so as to arise and be present in this moment.

Being mindful is also important because it enables you to develop a more conscious approach both to other people and the world around you. Greater self-awareness helps you to identify and recognize the triggers inside you that spark anger in relationships. Being more aware empowers you to notice the magnitude of your impact on others and how to make more positive and effective responses in your relationships.

Understanding Mindfulness

Mindfulness also referred to as awareness is always present, receptive, non-judging and observant of what is happening here and now. Becoming more mindful opens the door to a dimension of presence and stillness that is always near. As a human being, you can enter this dimension any moment thereby giving you the opportunity to be mindful of each thought, each step you take, each sound, smell, sensation or taste that you experience.

Since mindfulness is intricately linked to your existence, you constantly experience mindful moments even if you do not realize them to a lesser degree. An example of the moments when your mindfulness is in operation is when you notice the rushing sound of a truck or car passing nearby, the smell of food cooking or the touch of a gentle breeze against your face. The instant when the sensation makes contact with you, your brain transfers the signals deep into your consciousness so that you can understand the experience you are going through.

Mindfulness therefore is all about being aware of what is happening at the present moment. By placing a thought under the illuminating light of awareness, mindfulness opens a path for transformation and healing because it completely changes your relationship to your thoughts. For instance, when you are engaged in a conversation with someone, mindfulness can help keep you in the present so that you can hear what the other person is saying and know your own feelings and thoughts even better.

Scholarly Perspectives on Mindfulness

Scholarly definitions from some of the top mindful meditation teachers in the world help shed more light into the discipline and science of mindfulness.

Joseph Goldstein, a co-founder of the Insight Meditation Society defines mindfulness as the quality of paying full attention to the moment and opening to the truth of change. He went further to state that mindfulness is the quality of mind that notices what is present without judgment and interference.

Jon Kabat-Zinn, the celebrated creator of mindfulness-based stress reduction says that mindfulness is a moment-to-moment awareness. It is cultivated by deliberately paying attention to things we commonly never give a thought to. It is a systematic approach to the development of new forms of control and wisdom in our lives which are based on our inner capacities for paying attention, relaxation, insight and awareness.

Thich Nhat Hanh, a Zen teacher, author, poet and peace activist uses the term mindfulness to refer to the keeping of your consciousness alive to the present reality.

Sharon Salzberg, a co-founder of the Insight Meditation Society says mindfulness helps us get better at seeing the difference between what is happening and the stories we tell ourselves about what is happening, stories that get in the way of direct experience.

Mindfulness and Meditation

As human beings, we have a vast territory of awareness available to us. By practicing mindfulness, you can appropriate the benefits of that territory to your own life. Being mindful even for a single step or breath moves you deeper into the present moment and farther down the path of awareness. Practicing mindfulness offers you the much envied opportunity of discovering and experiencing the spaciousness and inner stillness as well as the simplicity and ease of living everyday that is your natural heritage.

There are a variety of meditation methods that can help strengthen your capacity to be mindful, increase your ability to sustain attention on a focal point and expand your capacity to remain present to any life experience with a non-judging and open attitude. Meditation simply refers to the practice of paying attention in a certain way for a particular purpose. It is both an art and a skill. The skills of meditation involve attention, intention and maintenance of a non-judging attitude. As an art, mediation involves self-transformation.

Christina Feldman, the meditation teacher, outlined a number of core principles that underlie all meditative disciplines:

- Attention - This refers to the means of establishing yourself in the present moment.

- Awareness - This is the development of a consciousness that is unburdened, light, sensitive and clear. It provides a still and intuitive inner environment.

- Understanding – This is the product of your immediate perception of both your inner and outer worlds. By developing understanding through meditation, you gain access to the possibility of traveling new pathways in your life that are part of the deepening tapestry of wisdom.

- Compassion - This is a fundamental principle of meditation. It brings out the selflessness and non-narcissistic nature of meditation.

Meditation is therefore the art and practice of building skills for sustaining attention, developing an awareness that is clear and gaining enhanced self-understanding into how to live wisely. Meditation is also supported by compassion and kindness which are not only basic human qualities but also attributes that are present in each person who meditates. Irrespective of the method of meditation you choose, each of the principles discussed above is present to some degree.

Mindfulness meditation practices give you the opportunity to successfully manage stress and other negative emotions including anger by deepening your awareness of these emotions and the triggers behind them.

Core Attitudes and Skills that Support Mindfulness

There are three main skills that have been identified by teachers and researchers which when fully developed, help you to experience the full potential of your natural heritage for being mindful. These skills are:

- Intention - This precedes every action you take whether consciously or unconsciously. You must intend to be mindful to counteract the deep seated habits of inattention and absence from the present moment that are part of the human nature.

- Attention - This skill is critical and you should practice and develop it at every moment. You may have noticed through your own life experiences that attention sometimes moves away from the subject of focus. Attention is much more useful when it is sustained and flexible.

- Attitude - The attitude of non-judgment and acceptance of everything that comes your way at the present moment is a critical component in mindfulness practice. Cultivating an accepting and non-judging attitude will help you achieve much in life. The mental habits of judging and reactivity arise in the body and mind very quickly and sweep you away into criticizing and blaming others

The attitude skill has many dimensions and expressions meaning you have a constellation of possibilities for deepening your skill of being aware and in the present. Jon Kabat-Zinn summarized 7 cores attitudes that are central in the practice of mindfulness. These are: non-judging, non-striving, trust, patience, acceptance, letting go, and beginners mind.

Scientific Evidence and Research Support for Mindfulness Practice

When your hostility and anger are chronically out of control or unmanaged, they can have harmful and fatal effects. In order to manage anger, you have to learn how to manage stress, how to perceive and relate to other people, and changing the attitudes and beliefs you hold about yourself and others. Practicing mindfulness can help you in gaining tremendous improvements in each of these areas.

According to research on mindfulness, the practice can help you deal with the toxic effects and triggers of anger as well as other difficult emotions inside you. In some of the studies done (Grossman et al; 2004; Baer 2003; Brown, Ryan, and Creswell 2007), mindfulness practice was shown to reduce the negative impact of stress on your health.

Mindfulness also helps to develop better understanding of other people and our capacity for empathy. Carson et al; 2004 conducted a research with couples who were practicing mindfulness. The results showed a significant improvement in relationship satisfaction, increased feelings of relatedness and acceptance of each other.

Practicing mindfulness helps you to grow self-awareness as well as thinking habits that influence your sense of self-worth and self-concept. In one of the research studies, it was discovered by simply being in a mindful state even momentarily, you stand a greater opportunity to experience a deeper sense of wellbeing.

As you practice mindfulness, remember that it is a universal possibility for every person. It also enables you to enter a dimension of life that provides real freedom from destructive emotions such as anger and the damaging effect of chronic stress.

2: Understanding your Anger

It is impossible to enter into any world for which you do not know its language – Ludwig Wittgenstein.

All of us live in the present moment, whatever event unfolds in our lives it is here and now. The past is simply but a memory that is happening in the present moment while the future is something that has yet to happen but we can imagine it or plan it now. Patterns of anger require an expenditure of energy by both your body and mind. The circuits and connections through which these energies flow can become extremely powerful if you allow anger to continue running unmanaged.

Since the energies that power the patterns of anger and related feelings in you have become a habit, you can refer to them as habit energies. If you want to take back control of your life from the habit energies of irritation, anger, judgments, hatred, rage and blame, it is important to understand accurately the nature of these energies, how they arise in the present moment, and the factors that trigger and sustain them every time they appear.

It is vitally important to reclaim your life from destructive emotions including anger. Paul Ekman, a renowned researcher in human emotions observed that it requires great effort to be able to restrain yourself from responding to anger with anger. One of the main problems people face with anger is the fact that it arises so quickly that they do not see it coming. Before you realize it, the rage and heat of anger is already burning in and around you. Anger drives us to act physically or verbally in ways that are harmful both immediately and overtime.

According to research evidence, people are simply not aware that their feelings amount to anger due to a lack of awareness of the present moment. There are lots of reasons that explain this lack of awareness but the good news is that with insight, these reasons can be understood and overcome.

One of the most obvious yet critical aspects of anger is that it occurs in the present moment. Anytime you experience anger, your sensations and angry thoughts arise and move through the present moment.

What is Anger?

Human beings naturally experience intense combinations of physical and mental events known as emotions. Anger is one of the basic human emotions. There is a notable consensus among emotion psychologists and researchers that anger is an integrated mind-body experience. This means anger involves thoughts, feelings and sensations in your body.

According to Joseph LeDoux, a researcher studying the brain mechanisms underlying emotions, notes that our memory systems have a part called working memory that allows us to know that here and now is here and it is happening right now. According to him, the state of mind or emotion you experience in this moment is the emotional information entering and being delivered into your working memory. The key components of this emotional information streaming in are the sensations happening in your body and the thoughts in your mind.

For instance, if you feel angry during a conversation with a person, the thoughts of anger are as a result of the thoughts you have concerning the conversation. The stream of body sensations and thoughts are the emotional information that is feeding your working memory and creating the emotional present for you.

Anger management experts concur with this approach of thoughts and body sensations and usually structure their anger intervention techniques to help their clients become more focused on the thought patterns and their bodily experience of anger. According to experts and teachers of mindfulness, emotions such as anger compromise basic building blocks including body sensation and thoughts. According to Joseph Goldstein, emotions are complex because they involve thoughts, images, moods and feelings in the body. Following years of reviewing psychological research, Ray Rosenman made a conclusion that perception of an event determines the emotional response and the psycho-physiological consequences.

Anger is a cognitive process associated with personal appraisal and interpretation. The key to understanding and managing anger lies in the recognition that a state of bodily arousal is present, the nature of your perception to the situation, and knowledge of the thoughts and inner narrative you generate about the perception. Depending on the thoughts that follow and the meaning you assign to the situation, the unfolding experience of anger can either cool down or heat up.

Anger is Thoughts plus Sensations

Assume you are driving or even walking and someone abruptly blocks the way; it is natural to feel irritated or angry. After the person goes away, a number of things may run through your mind and body. By chaining your thoughts, that is, adding more and more thoughts to the original emotion of anger, you are in essence feeding your feelings of anger and internal upset. You may find yourself gradually feeling the growing anger which may direct you to hurt the other person.

On the contrary, you can simply shake your head and dismiss the inconvenience that the person caused you. When you do this, there is no chaining of thoughts that happen and your inner fire of anger lacks the ongoing fuel to power it. When faced with anger, you can decide to intentionally respond with compassion as this is the healthier way of doing things. To achieve this, you must first acknowledge your feeling of anger and gradually shift your inner story to focusing on the positive instead of condemning the acts of the other person.

Learning how to uncouple your thought train responsible for carrying your anger on and on, you will find peace of mind within yourself. If you observe carefully, you will find that your own runaway thought train is the one feeding your angry feelings and sustaining the animosity you feel towards the other party. Mathew Ricard noted that anger is an expression of animosity towards the other person.

Developing a capacity to recognize and respond to sensations and thoughts that cause and sustain anger is absolutely critical in helping you regain control of your life. Even in the changing winds of experiences blowing through the present moment in your life, you will become unshakable and steady.

The Functions of Anger

Anger serves a number of purposes in humans and that is why it is so common and quick to arise in each one of us. The basic functions of anger are protection and survival.

Anger for Survival

Human beings have evolved amidst dangers from starvation, diseases and predators. Our biology has also evolved and more so then our brain and nervous system. In the face of danger, it is advantageous for people to cooperate within their own groups and be aggressive towards others. The groups that had greater cooperation ended up being more successful at aggression. Aggression is normally a response to threats and includes subtle feelings of anxiety and unease.

Anger for Protection

Whenever you sense danger, your body and mind immediately goes into a freezing-fight-or-flight mode to protect you from harm. The fight or flight mode gives the indication that you are ready to defend yourself by either fleeing or fighting the perceived danger. Freezing on the other hand is a state of paralysis that the body uses to avoid being harmed.

Anger as a Barrier against Unwanted Thoughts and Feelings

Anger can protect you from external feelings that you do not necessarily want to experience. Whenever you go through disturbing thoughts and feelings, anger may arise to protect you. This is psychologically referred to as defensive anger because it defends you from experiencing disturbing feelings and inner thoughts.

The defensive anger can immediately pop up even before realizing the presence of unpleasant or disturbing thoughts inside of you. To this end, it can be said that defensive anger is excellent in defending you from feeling anything strange and unpleasant. However, the tricky part is that by not acknowledging the unpleasant feelings and thoughts, you give them an opportunity to grow inside you. When unpleasant feelings are suppressed or denied for a long time, they may get stronger and come back with a vengeance when you least expect it.

Response to Obstacles

The function of anger is to remove whatever interferences we are experiencing. The anger response has a built-in impulse to remove the obstacle that is barricading your way.

In Buddhism, there are five common hindrances or obstacles to the meditation practice. These hindrances are viewed as filters or energies that distort our moment-by-moment relationship to the experiences unfolding in our lives. The influence of any hindrance energy immediately spreads to our interior experiences of feelings, thoughts and body sensations. It colors our perceptions and dictates how we interact with others. These 5 hindrances are desire, aversion and ill-will, sloth and torpor, restlessness, and doubt. These hindrances are not confined to Buddhism as a religion but rather are experienced by every human being.

When anger strikes, something happens in our body and mind. As human beings, we are equipped with an alarm system that helps us to combat and evade threats to survive. The nervous system plays a critical role in your anger response through your senses. There is a release of hormones and other complex reactions in your body that increase your odds of survival and enables you to fight, flee or freeze.

Therefore, if you want to control your anger, you must learn how to recognize when it is present in your life. You must understand that anger can take on many faces and can appear as dislike, aversion or ill-will to what is present.

3: How to Objectively Approach Anger

When you become mindful, the world and everything in it will appear differently. Mindfulness is all about becoming aware of what is happening here and now. It opens another dimension in your life and gives you the opportunity to expand your level of awareness which gives you a totally different and more positive relationship towards yourself and others.

Entering into this mindfulness-based dimension will give you a wide range of choices. It will also give you certain wisdom about yourself that is true and resonates with your healthiest and deepest values that no one can shake. Practicing mindfulness can be quite challenging. This chapter will usher you into the practice of mindfulness and how you can objectively approach anger through it.

Mindfulness Can Observe Your Anger

The perspective of mindfulness is that everything including anger happens in the present moment. Anger is an experience that is rooted deep into your sense of your personal identity and depends on feelings, thoughts and sensations. This means that mindfulness can help you take control of your life from anger as long as you bring it into your inner life. Your inner life simply refers to the stream of interior experiences that flow through your sensations and senses. Your sensory texture and mental activity changes moment by moment. It is made up of your feelings and your thoughts.

From the view of mindfulness, your inner life consists of moment by moment experiences of emotions such as anger, thinking, and the flow of information into your senses. These experiences are intimate, personal and keep on changing hence they do not have a permanent identity. A careful observation of anger reveals that it is a temporal condition without a defining identity. It can be understood, controlled, and transformed through radical and powerful relationships.

Approaching anger mindfully requires that you commit to building a relationship with anger rather than throwing in the towel and labeling yourself as a victim of it. Adopting a right approach to anger will switch your attention and curiosity towards the experience of anger and its various related expressions.

Approaching anger skillfully requires that you develop the necessary skills to be mindful of your anger whenever it appears. These skills include a strong intention to become more aware of your anger, stopping and paying attention to each moment even when the emotions are distracting and upsetting, and keeping a welcoming attitude to whatever is unfolding in your awareness.

The ability to recognize and embrace emotional experiences irrespective of how intense they are is a skill that can be developed. When the events that are causing anger changes, there is tendency to have a painful memory of it. As human beings, we are wired to selectively remember the signals and signs associated with an alarming situation much more easily than the memory of pleasant or good things. This selective recall of unpleasant and negative experiences is known as negative bias.

Mindful attention makes it clear that the situations or conditions that cause anger or other emotional experience are changing temporarily. By practicing mindfulness, you can be more present whenever the experience happen as well as recognize how it changes color and shape. This will in turn give you the opportunity to respond wisely whenever the memory of the event comes back.

Ways to Exercise a Mindful Approach

There are lots of ways you can use to approach your anger mindfully. Each of these methods emphasizes a particular meditative or reflective focus. These approaches are used by experts in meditation and those offering mindfulness-based interventions. They are effective and easy to learn.

Stopping and Seeing

As previously discussed, human beings are wired for protection and self-defense. This is why in times of strong emotion such as anger, the sensations and thoughts arise and sweep us very quickly. In order to disentangle yourself from the sticky web of angry emotions, it is important to stop and look more closely so you are aware of what is happening. There are many meditative practices that use mindfulness to help you disentangle your over-identification with your inner stream of thoughts and sensations. These practices will ultimately enable you to have an accurate focus of attention to what is happening.

Compassion and Kindness

One of the impacts of anger is to feel lonely, isolated and disconnected from the rest. This distorted view can be rectified if you desire. You can choose a meditation practice that cultivates the quality of compassion or kindness so as to support the mindfulness skill of maintaining a welcoming and non-judging attitude. Knowing how to approach anger mindfully by way of finding and resting in your inborn capacity for goodness can be very helpful.

Taking a Wise View

Taking a wise view of what anger can equip and inform your response when the intense emotion of anger storms over you. Just like a rainbow, anger changes constantly. Every time you observe the experience of anger mindfully, you will notice that what you thought was anger is a complex formation of elements that appear in the present moment.

According to the structural model of anger, fear lies beneath anger and beneath fear is a fixed belief. These beliefs are the conditions that nurture your anger. Using the wise view approach to anger, you will notice that anger is built on judgmental thoughts that are often untrue. When you notice the presence of judging thoughts that are mere fabrication, you will not be moved by them nor will you act upon them.

You can comfortably approach and take control of anger using any of the above ways. They will help you escape over-identification through cultivation of kindness and compassion towards yourself as well as others.

As a mindfulness practice of finding anger in your body, you should take a deliberate stand to stop and pay attention whenever you receive signals of anger. Give yourself a chance to understand your experience of anger and stabilize it without judging anyone. Feel the sensations in different areas of your body, stay observant and disentangle the stream of anger in you. Remember as you practice mindfulness, the world around you will become more interesting, vivid and alive. This will help you calm your angry mind.

4: Calming Your Anger through Mental and Body Stability

If you want to control anger as well as other strong emotions, you need to take a view from the present moment. The advantage with this view is that it is centered in the present moment and recognizes that anything that happens; happens within the present context. Your thought processes, sensations and feelings in your body, even the most intense emotions, such as anger always arise, unfold and fade in the present moment.

When you are remembering the past or planning for your future, the associations, emotions and thoughts involved change, arise and move in and out of the present moment through the ever changing brain patterns and neural activity.

The fate of anger just like any emotion depends upon the conditions in the present moment that sustains the feelings. For instance, if you are waiting for a service and you become impatient because of the slow moving line at the checkout, your anger is likely to grow in direct proportion to the degree that you keep judging and sulking inside. Repeating the chain of angry words and thoughts fuels your anger and your aggravation and suffering will continue to grow as you advance towards the checkout counter.

In any given situation, the length of time you remain angry is directly proportional to the duration in which you remain caught in the river of angry thoughts. The more you continue to feed your anger the more it will blossom. Therefore, learning to recognize the presence of angry energy in your mind and body and knowing how to disentangle yourself is crucial. It is like learning a life-saving skill.

This chapter introduces you to 5 meditation practices that will help you build and strengthen your skills so that you can steady yourself even when the storm of anger threatens you.

The Brake of Mindfulness

As pointed out earlier, we all have a natural capacity to notice events happening in the present. This is a powerful brake on the runaway train of anger. Everyone longs for a simpler life where we can rest in the stillness and space that allows us to touch our inner rhythms and the world around us in a much more intimate and authentic way. Uncontrolled anger is often frustrating and keeps us from realizing the benefits that come with a deeper connection between ourselves and the world.

Bringing mindfulness can add a new dimension in your life that will help you rediscover the vast landscape of awareness. As a practice, each moment you notice irritation or anger, remember to stop and step back. You should not judge yourself for the feeling of anger; instead you should practice the qualities of patience and non-judgment towards yourself. Bringing mindfulness to the present makes you step out from the situation you are in for a moment so that you can shift your attention to a more productive response to your anger.

Practice Mindful Breathing

Your body and your mind are dynamically interactive and interconnected moment by moment. This is why it is difficult for them to be separated. You will notice that when thoughts of anger arise in your mind, they are almost immediately translated into your body for action. Your mind and your body understand how to generate feelings of well-being that will help you to balance the mental and physical intensities of freeze-fight-or-flight.

Knowing how to signal your mind and body to shift into feelings of well-being even in moments of anger can help you to relax and calm down. It is one of the most important skills of self-care and personal stress management. When your feelings ease, your capacity to see clearly greatly increases and you will experience greater degree of presence in every moment.

When practicing meditation, you should remind yourself of the core attitudes of mindfulness practice – not judging and not striving. Mindful breathing is much more than the ease that it brings. It helps you to be in the present moment so you may be aware, open and be unshakable.

Returning Your Mind to the Present

Your body always lives in the present but your mind spends a lot of time wandering. Oftentimes it is preoccupied with regrets and memories of the past and anxieties and worries of the future. Learning to return your attention and sustaining it can help you unite your mind and body so that both can live in the present moment.

If you want to calm your angry mind, you have to notice first where it has gone, then return it to the present moment. For instance, instead of becoming lost in anger or upset in thoughts, you should practice mindfulness of your body. The good news is that irrespective of the activity you are in, you can practice mindfulness. Learning to inhabit your body with awareness is an important element for self-care, overall healing, building happier and richer life, as well as for growing emotional intelligence.

Gathering the Courage to Let it Be

Human beings are little more complex because they are wired to survive any experience of painful thoughts. It can easily activate a burning desire to escape or change what is happening in the present moment. The urge to change something can be so strong that it causes anger and irritation. It is a fact that many times your ability to change things is either limited or non-existent.

By gathering the courage to let it be, you can comfortably step out of the reactive and rapid cycle of frustration that arises when you realize there is almost nothing you can do to change a particular situation. Through this practice of meditation, you can draw on your natural capacity for mindfulness and resting upon the qualities of acceptance and courage to access your capacity for equanimity. This will help you to allow things to take their natural course at least for the moment.

Your mind uses memories and fear of past pain, disappointments and failure to scare you away from stopping and examining yourself. By having faith and trusting yourself that you have what it takes, you can feel the strength of courage, equanimity and acceptance to confront your fearful thoughts. This empowerment you get from realization cannot be snatched away from you. Remember, courage does not mean the absence of fear but rather the capacity to stand firm in the face of fear.

Balancing the Feelings of Fear

According to the structure of anger, the topmost layer is anger, then beneath it is fear and the foundation of it all is belief systems. Once you realize that fear underlies all the thoughts and feelings of anger, it is possible to address it much more directly. Through loving-kindness mediation, you can learn how to powerfully balance your feelings of fear.

Loving-kindness meditation is simply resting on your natural human capacity for friendliness, kindness and compassion and using that as the foundation to shift out of your painful and isolating mental tendencies. According to the stories written about Buddha, it is said that he taught loving-kindness meditation to all his nuns and monks as the antidote to fear.

Modern psychology has shown the existence of correlation between meditation practices founded in loving-kindness and better results in terms of health, happiness and well-being. Loving-kindness can therefore be useful in gaining stability during a storm of rage or when facing challenges of a frightening situation.

Remember, practicing mindfulness can enable you apply the brakes to anger, find peace, and discover your courage and strength as well as understanding through compassion and kindness.

5: Calming Your Anger through Compassion

Mother Teresa once said *"In this life, we cannot do great things. We can only do small things with great love."* At one point or another, each one of us must have experienced a situation where a perfect stranger or friend was in pain and you had to rush to help them. This is compassion. According to social scientists, compassion is an innate goodness of heart that recognizes the pain of another person and the urge to do something to help relieve the pain.

The Concept of Compassion

As human beings, we have nervous systems and brains that arc selectively wired for compassion. There are connections between certain neurons and regions in our brain that support social intuition which is a key dimension of our emotional life. We also have neural and psychological systems that help us to nurture our children, bond with mates and come together as a community for a common cause.

Research reveals the existence of a core network of connections in the lower and middle regions of our brains that integrate multiple, emotional and social capabilities. Extending compassion to yourself

(self-compassion) is very important for your physical and mental health. It helps strengthen resilience, lower stress hormones and reduce toxic self-criticism. This chapter opens up in an attempt to explore your built-in capacity to experience, access and nurture compassion.

Compassion is not a project into some future moment or a quality to idealize, rather compassion is a response to any moment of confusion, pain and suffering either in another person or in you. Turning to compassion is not as difficult and it does not require you to become a saint or a better person than you already are. Just believe in yourself that you have everything you need within you to be compassionate.

Compassion is a crucial resource that you can use in controlling your anger. Ancient meditation, spiritual teachings and modern science have found the practice of compassion to be a profound vehicle for transformation and enjoyment of much healthier lives. Through compassion, you can activate your brain and body systems to help you move from old habit patterns to a more expanded and accurate perception of your connections with others. This expanded and more generous feeling within you helps to broaden and build your capacity for staying present with less rejection and anger.

Discovering the Power of Self-Compassion

Psychologists and researchers agree that most people turn to be their own worst critics. Self-critical tendencies are harmful to your health and contribute to distorted and inaccurate views of yourself as not valuable or worthy. These views deny your inherent goodness and worth as a person and form a ripe ground to grow and sustain destructive and chronic feeling of fear and anger.

Dr. Kristin Neff, a pioneering researcher in self-compassion established that self-compassion is crucial to living a happier and productive life. According to her, compassion consists of three main components:

Self-Kindness

This is the practice of actively comforting ourselves each moment we feel pain.

Common Humanity

This is the recognition of our connection with other people including the fact that all of us experience aging, pain, sickness as well as death.

Mindfulness

This refers to the capacity to hold our experience in a balanced awareness instead of ignoring or exaggerating our pain.

As you practice discovering self-compassion, take a moment and appreciate each part of your body from the soles of your feet to the crown of your head. By appreciating yourself, you become much more aware of how important each part of you is and how amazing you are as a person.

The Interconnectedness of Pain and Compassion

Anger and fear are in close proximity to compassion. The feelings of anger or fear that arise within you can block the feeling of compassion for others. This interference with your capacity for compassion makes you feel separate and perhaps alienated from the situation and the person in pain.

According to teachers of meditation, it is critically important to acknowledge and not deny the truth and the causes of suffering and pain that we experience. Our willingness to turn towards our pain and seek to understand it can give us a pathway to discovering a different relationship to the pain we are experiencing. We will be able to include the pain in awareness and embrace it with compassion. The moment you realize that the pain in you has the same qualities and causes as the pain in another person, you will experience greater compassion for other people. Anytime you feel disconnected or isolated from others, you should pause for a moment to acknowledge and investigate those feelings with mindful attention and compassion.

Directions for Forgiveness

Resentment is the sense of indignation or hurt that comes from feeling offended or injured. Resentment comes from the Latin word meaning to feel again. To be indignant means to express feelings of scorn or anger especially at another person who has been ungrateful or unjust. The roots of indignant mean not worthy. Indignation and resentment can fuel chronic feelings of blame and anger.

As human beings, we go through events in life that arouse feelings of resentment and at times indignation. The hurt we experience in our relationships or lives come when another person intends to harm us. Whether intentional or non-intentional, the acts of others that hurt us can fuel the feelings of resentment every time we think about the particular event. Unmanaged and chronically carried resentment requires a little spark to explode into the present moment and completely distort our experience of what is here and now.

It is common to feel resentment towards other people but we often forget that our own actions could have also hurt other people and may make them feel resentment towards us. The good news is that resentment and indignation can be remedied through forgiveness. Forgiveness is simply defined as the end of resentment. By being aware of the present, you give yourself an opportunity to end resentment and cultivate qualities of kindness and compassion.

Sorrow, Kindness and Equanimity

Pain when coupled with the feelings of vulnerability and helplessness can easily sermon anger and fear. In turn, these energies take us away from the present and interfere with our response of compassion. However, the choice to respond to any pain is always present and we can cultivate and strengthen our capacity to make a better choice. Equanimity is a spacious stillness of the mind and a radiant calm that enables us to be present fully with all changing experiences that constitute our world. As we slowly learn to accept the truth of change and develop the ability to let go, our equanimity deepens.

There is a need to cultivate a balance between compassion which is the tenderness of our hearts in response to suffering and anger, and equanimity which is the spacious stillness that makes us accept things as they are. When we attain this balance, we can successfully remain present and deeply in touch with any instance of sorrow and pain that we face. Responding with kindness and not anger can help bring profound positive consequences for every person involved. Phrases that acknowledge limits and promote peacefulness can be used to cultivate the quality of equanimity.

Engaging in practices focused on compassion, kindness and equanimity can help you reconnect with the goodness of heart that is in every human being.

6: Tapping into Wisdom to Calm Your Anger

In our busy lives as human beings, we find ourselves carried away by strong and changing inner currents of strong emotions such as anger, thoughts and intense body sensations. Each of the inner currents is itself caused by a number of conditions that are constantly changing in the present moment. Your inner atmospheric conditions of body and mind include your cognitions, physical status, and the constant stream of information that comes through your senses every time you interact with other people.

These elements combine to form powerful inner currents that have the capacity to carry you forward into more emotions and thoughts as well as actions. By watching closely and mindfully, you can observe your body sensations forming around your thoughts. You watch how your inner reactions to the world outside evoke judgments that activate strong reactive sensations and demanding thoughts in your mind. The flow of experience through your body and mind shifts and so are the ways in which you perceive the world around you.

For instance, as you walk down the street, you may have experienced a warm feeling even towards a perfect stranger. When you look at the moments before you met this person, you will realize that you were feeling happy and at ease. On the other hand, if you feed your mind with angry thoughts, you will feel threatened by everybody around you, especially strangers.

Developing awareness and having a more accurate understanding can immensely benefit us and lead us toward a more fulfilling life that is less dominated by the toxicity of hostility and chronic anger.

When we experience strong emotions such as anger, we must understand that we are not failures because of what we feel. Rather, being angry is part of our human experience. However, the degree to which we are aware of this strong emotion, the meaning we assign to it and the relationship we forge with it makes a whole lot of difference in how we fashion our response.

When His Holiness the Dalai Lama was addressing a group of enthusiasts after being awarded the Nobel Peace Prize, someone asked him whether he gets angry. He said that at times things happen in our lives that are not part of our original plan and anger rises in us. However, he was quick to point out that anger does not have to be a problem. This chapter will help you in changing your experience of anger through wisdom and understanding.

When you identify the conditions that support your anger, the emotional and mental habits that sustain anger, fear, blame, scorn and hostility will lose their power over you.

Anger as a Temporal Condition

You can be easily carried in the whirlwind of angry emotions if you forget that anger like all other emotions is not permanent. Anger is a condition that arises when other non-anger elements that support it are present. Focusing your attention on anger and noticing how it changes, you can gradually see the truth that anger is only temporary. This can be a source of strength for you when anger appears again momentarily in the future. Remember that even in the heat of anger, you can maintain emotional stability.

The Cloud of Anger

Each one of us had an opportunity to watch the clouds in the sky. Have you ever realized or considered that a cloud is made up of elements and conditions that are not in themselves clouds? Clouds of every kind appear but they only do so when there are conditions that support them. From science, you may know that these conditions are temperature, moisture, pressure and light. None of these conditions is a cloud in its own capacity; however, they have to be together for cloud to form. When these conditions are not present, there is no cloud and therefore nothing to see.

In the same way, a shoe is a name we sign to something that is made of certain materials that have qualities of feel, color, shape, durability and size which serve a number of functions. Just like the cloud, the shoe is made up of non-shoe elements.

For something to exist a number of elements have to come up. It gives you a wise and radical shift to look at your anger again. Anger, like a cloud is a temporarily coming together of particular conditions.

Getting to know the different conditions necessary for your cloud of anger to appear can help you re-identify, uncouple and escape from any angry feelings that may otherwise hijack you.

Stop Feeding Your Anger

One useful approach of calming your anger is to identify the constituting elements and take some of them away. This effectively removes the props that sustain your anger. In moments of anger, the most important question to ask yourself is – what fuels my anger? Most often than not, we tend to blame others for our anger. This is an incorrect understanding and a response that is not helpful because we have limited, if any control over the actions of other people.

If someone made you angry or at least you have a reason to believe so, you cannot continue living in anger or irritation waiting for them to change. Blame is an unconscious form of resistance to the way the world appears to us and to our own pain. Most times we do not realize how we push back and protest against what we feel inside of us or in the world around us.

Through mindfulness, you can observe your pain and your resistance to it. You will discover that pain is inevitable in our lives but the suffering that results depends on our resistance whenever the pain arises. It is therefore clear that blame and resistance to pain can fuel anger but our lack of self-awareness is the real culprit.

The pain we experience in our lives is not so much in the circumstances that we face but in the response and relationship we take to what is happening. By growing self-awareness of what is happening around us, we can comfortably calm our angry minds. You have power within your own intelligence and goodness to help you ease the resistance and eliminate some of the fuel that is responsible for your anger.

Confronting Your Obstacles

Almost everyone loves the idea of being free. The freedom to do what you like, to come and go, to experience whatever you want with your body and many other things. Most people experience times when their minds feel caged and devoid of freedom. For instance, you may be occupied doing a task and your mind suddenly wonders with the desire to do something else that is more pleasant. This desire diminishes your effectiveness in whatever it is that you are doing.

Freedom in your mind and body can be lost to feelings of restlessness in the form of agitation. Restlessness can keep you away from settling into something that you are trying hard to do. Doubting thoughts can be persuasive and intimidating and can stimulate feelings of worry and anxiety. The desire for something else, fatigue, restlessness, doubt and aversion can hinder you from living freely and happily because they conquer your mind and influence your body. Aversion and ill-will are responsible for directly feeding your feelings and thoughts of anger. Unfortunately, these hindrances are very common in our lives. To overcome them, you need to focus your attention directly onto the hindrances and use your awareness to illuminate them. This makes it easy for you to shift your relationship and hence overcome the obstacles to your freedom.

To calm your anger, you also need to build and broaden your resilience and your response capacity to anger. When life confronts you with difficult challenges, irritation, annoyances and other unpleasant experiences, it can be very difficult. Research in psychology has shown that intentional cultivation of positivity can have powerful benefits. Some of the positive emotions that you should focus on include gratitude, joy, serenity, hope, interest, amusement, love and inspiration.

Nourishing positivity within you can help in broadening your inner resources to help you cope with strong emotions such as anger. Nourishing positivity helps to strengthen your capacity to meet difficult moments with interest and compassion rather than reactively going to war with what is happening around you.

7: Belonging and Interconnection

Anger is a master illusionist. Scornful, hostile or angry feelings can trick you into believing that you are permanently isolated from other people around you. When your thoughts are filled with dislike and resentment for others, you may be easily convinced that no one respects, sees or even hears you. As a matter of fact, the belief that you are in isolation can make you project your anger onto others even if they have not done anything to harm you.

The voices of anger deep inside you can deceive you and obscure your recognition of your role and true place in the web of life. Distortions that come from an angry mind can effectively block your conscious perception of the connection you have with others. They can also cloud your sensitivity to the interconnection and interdependency of all living things.

Becoming aware of your present, you will slowly disengage from isolation and alienation to anger. Mindfulness reminds us that we belong in this life and invites us to befriend our feelings of self-doubt, alienation, unworthiness as well as the anger that drives them. Through mindfulness, you can gain access to a new dimension that is not limited by thoughts and sensations of anger. You will remain steady and mindfully aware of every changing thought or feeling of isolation and separation as it happens. This will in turn free you from the imprisonment that thoughts of anger can drive you into.

Irrespective of their source, feelings of loneliness and isolation are misperceptions and distortions of our situations as human beings.

A Scientific View of Relationships

According to modern neuroscience, we all have systems in our mind and body which are constantly interacting to promote empathy, understanding and concern for one another. According to this research, human beings must cooperate in order to survive; cooperation is more important to survival compared to aggression.

Daniel J. Siegel, an expert in interpersonal neurobiology indicated that relationships are the sharing of information and energy flow. Integrative communication refers to the sharing of information and energy where each individual's internal world is respected and allowed to be differentiated. Through integrative communication, development of healthy relationships can take place.

For instance, when you see someone who is sad, your various brain circuits related to memories, emotions and self-awareness become activated.

This will cause you to experience similar feelings and sooner than later, you will begin to develop a deeper sense of communication and identification with the other party. Your relationship with the other person becomes information-filled and more empathetic. This is because of the power behind the interpersonal neurobiology circuits present in all of us.

In applying the scientific interpretation of what constitutes our sense of self can be very instrumental, particularly in times when anger or ill-will, have taken over your emotions. Every time your emotions are painful and your thoughts of isolation become louder and more convincing, remember that your feelings of loneliness, pain and isolation are not permanent. Instead, you are constantly being upheld, formed and made to feel more solid by information and energy streams, thoughts and feelings that are briefly present, flowing and always changing within you.

Deep inside, you can help transform the pain that sustains your anger. When you are afraid, angry, stuck and feeling alone, becoming aware and compassionate can help you to recognize that you belong in this moment and no one can fall out of the universe.

When you look closely enough, you may notice the changing, complex and rich tapestry that forms reality in every moment of your life. The long threads of countless relationships and people, and moments of experience, all contribute to the beautiful particularity making you the person you are moment by moment.

If your attention is steady enough, you will be able to distinguish some of the threads that make this tapestry and observe the impact that people or places you experienced long ago have on your present moment. For instance, the smell of certain food brings back the memories of the times or holidays you had when you were growing up. The smell of the food may either bring good memories or summon painful feelings and memories of anxiety.

In whichever way, the fact remains that the way your mind reacts contribute and shape your experience as you relate with people in this very moment. If you wish to heal and transform your life into a happier one, you must manage the relationship that your past memories have with your present experience.

Anger Distracts and Blinds You

Feelings of anger and other emotive expressions of aversion and ill-will can blind us to the relationships connections and reality that is present. Feeling angry sustains a reaction in body and mind which produces a state of hyper-arousal. The inner thoughts and perceptions fueled by anger can distract and create an external target or focus for the anger. This in turn strengths and sustains the subjective feeling of being alone and isolated. These complex and anger-driven experiences will blind and distract you from the present moment.

Anger Distorts Your Perception of Other People

When you are angry at the present moment, it's very easy to misinterpret and misunderstand other people. For instance, when you are fuming about an incident at your workplace and someone makes a comment when you return home, even if it's not necessarily about you, chances of you personalizing the comment are very high.

When you are filled with anger, you may become super sensitive to even simple requests from family or friends. When you are angry, you risk falling into a self-focused narrative about how everybody disrespects you and take you for granted.

Anger Isolates

When an angry person yells at you or someone close to you raises their voice in a critical manner to something you have said or done, there should be a tendency for you to get away from that person as soon as possible.

People who are chronically angry, judgmental and overly critical end up feeling socially isolated because through their own criticisms and insensitivity, they have pushed others away.

Anger Distorts Self-Awareness

Anger projected onto others serves as an effective defense against painful feelings that you may be experiencing. Beneath your feelings of anger is fear as well as untrue and harsh beliefs about yourself and others. When angry feelings direct the blame outward onto situations or other people, your awareness and experience of yourself in that very moment is likely to be ignored and distorted.

Chronic feelings of ill-will and anger are turned both on yourself as well as others. When your inner voices and narratives are overly critical, there is very little space left for self-care or self-compassion. Whenever denial of pain, upset and fatigue are your first line of response to those painful feelings, the result is a damaging disconnection and blindness from your own body and feelings. The moment you begin to understand the belief of unworthiness that is upholding your fear, you will gradually start to heal and allow yourself to trust again in the basic truth of your own value and connections to life.

How to Correct Anger Distortions

Every distortion created by anger can be corrected. It is possible to disentangle from the feelings of alienation and delusion of isolation and experience the beauty of interconnection in any moment.

Life is only available in this moment. Because anger thrives on energies of pain-filled inner narratives, critical thoughts and negative meanings, it distracts and obscures you from the present moment and your treasured sense of belonging to life.

Anger, together with feelings of ill-will can take you into your past and future with painful narratives and critical thoughts. Anger often uses "should have and should have not's" as well as blaming judgments to survive. In real sense, anger hijacks you by filling the present moment with fears, memories about the past, and evokes intense mental and body reactions.

When we are absorbed in a self-centered perspective and holding defensively to a particular opinion or idea, we become limited in our ability to see the much larger content or to understand the position of other people with whom we disagree.

Becoming aware of your present moment will help you to interrupt that defensive, reactive energy of anger and create the possibility for a better outcome.

As human beings, there are so many ways in which we can be hurt. Such deep hurt is often the cornerstone of anger that continually brings together feelings of isolation and alienation. The good news is even old hurts can be healed! They do not have to be obstacles toward your joy or safety.

Seeing with New Eyes

The continuous interplay between our consciousness and interior life including our memories, body sensations, ideas, perceptions and beliefs, constitute our experience of being alive in the present moment. In countless and amazing ways, we interact with other people hence shaping and contributing to the unfolding reality of being alive.

Marcel Proust, a French novelist, made an interesting observation that having new eyes instead of seeking new landscapes is the most important element in any voyage of real discovery. The problem that many people have is viewing the world selectively through filters of sadness, pain, anger and fear which obscures everything that is present.

People often go to all lengths to distance themselves from painful, embarrassing or unwanted aspects of their behavior in the past. There is always a consequence for every attempt that you make to hide or deny a part of yourself that you feel shame, guilt or regret.

Remember, who you are at this moment is the result of your past accomplishments as well as your past failures. Your insights, blind spots, warts and beauty have contributed to you being the person you are today. If it were not for all those things, you would not be who you are today.

8: Lifestyle Changes for Anger Management

Having a healthy lifestyle is essential towards anger management. You can easily enhance your stress resistance levels by going through calculated lifestyle changes such as exercises, diet and therapy. Below is a discussion of some of the recommended lifestyle changes and how they impact your stress and anger management programs.

Exercise

As a stress and anger management technique, exercise is extremely important and very healthy for your overall health. When you engage in exercises, you are in essence shifting your focus from stressful and anger fueling events into workouts that improve your mood and boost your cardiac health.

Techniques such as Yoga or Tai chi combine the relaxation benefits of breathing and meditation while stretching and toning the muscles. During moments of anger, emotions fill your mind and as a result your body becomes tense. Through these exercises, your muscles have the opportunity to relax and hence normalize the blood flow. This empties your mind of angry thoughts and toxic emotions.

It is important that you start with a plan and execute it successfully. This will give you the feeling of accomplishment, mastery and control. Exercise, when shared with others can foster healthy relationships making it easy for you to appreciate and respect other people as well as yourself.

Cognitive-Behavioral Therapy

Therapy has been employed by professionals to combat various conditions involving mind and body. Anger is one of the excessive emotions that require expert attention and counseling hence the need for cognitive behavioral therapy. Compared to support groups, cognitive behavioral therapy is effective because it gives you the platform to voice out your concerns.

Typically, the therapists will take you through a small interview to understand your source of anger and stress. The therapist will then restructure priorities so you may change your response to the emotions you are facing. The activities that are putting a strain in your time, energy, and anger are all written down as well as the positive experiences that bring a sense of refreshment and accomplishment.

The therapist then carefully shifts the balance from the anger producing to anger reducing activities. This process is called restructuring of priorities. Elimination of stress and triggers of anger may not be feasible but through the right strategies, the impact can be reduced.

There are a number of relief options that can help ease your mind and to an extent calm your angry mind. Among these include:

- Listening to music – According to research, music soothes the mind and help in normalizing your blood pressure, anxiety levels as well as the heart rate. These are conditions present in your anger build up.
- Where the source of stress and anger is in your immediate surroundings, taking vacations may help to reenergize your mind. You will have a new environment to reconsider your thoughts and possibly find a way to coexist with others without necessarily being angry.
- Discussing your feelings – Most therapists encourage you to let out your feelings in an acceptable and responsible way. Feelings of anger that are hidden can cause frustration, depression, a sense of helplessness and even hostility. Expression of feelings however does not mean that you vent out your frustration

because doing so can irritate others and further widen the social gap caused by anger.

Relaxation and Other Methods

Anger is part of our lives and as such we need to develop methods that will promote a healthy response. Relaxation and natural unwinding is one of the responses that can ease anger and give you an opportunity to examine your inner self. Take time in the course of your busy schedule and just go somewhere quiet and peaceful or lock the door in your office and face a blank wall. This will help you to empty your toxic thoughts and emotions and embrace it with healthy ones.

Relaxation is effective because it brings your blood pressure down to normal level, releases muscle tension and helps in easing emotional strain. The response to relaxation is highly individualized although there is a general acceptance that indeed relaxation helps in easing stress, strain and anger.

Conclusion

Anger, just like a rainbow or a cloud depends on a myriad of conditions in order to manifest. It does not come from external sources but rather comes from within. It comes through events which triggers a complex set of conditions such as fears, beliefs, perceptions and physical reactions. Being aware of your anger and the factors that fuel it can build and broaden your resources. This will help you choose an appropriate response with compassion, understanding and knowledge of how to care for the pain masked by angry feelings.

Turning toward pain and anger with steady attention that is founded on wisdom and kindness can become your most trusted, wisest and effective response whenever anger rears its angry head. By trusting that you already have everything you need to combat anger and all its underlying emotions, you will have the confidence to radically shift your understanding of these emotions and the distorting power they have over your life.

Never act out the drama alone. Do not feel abandoned or isolated because in doing so, you will be denying the intimacy of your surroundings. May self-awareness in its entire expression blossom in your life and may you discover the dignity and courage to overcome your anger and transform your life for the better!